Keto Diet

Cookbook for

Beginners

A Simplified Guide To Make Easy And Delicious
Keto Diet Recipes

Juliana Diaz

the author responsible for any losses, direct or indirect, which are incurred as a result of the use of information contained within this document, including, but not limited to, — errors, omissions, or inaccuracies.

Table of Content

SMOOTHIES & BREAKFAST

Chaffles with Caramelized Apples and Yogurt

Serving: 2

Preparation Time: 5 minutes

Cooking Time: 10 minutes

Ingredients

- 1 tablespoon unsalted butter
- 1 tablespoon golden brown sugar
- 1 Granny Smith apple, cored and thinly sliced
- 1 pinch salt
- 2 whole-grain frozen waffles, toasted
- 1/2 cup mozzarella cheese, shredded
- 1/4 cup Yoplait® Original French Vanilla yogurt

Direction

1. Melt the butter in a large skillet over medium-high heat until starting to brown. Add mozzarella cheese and stir well.

2. Add the sugar, apple slices and salt and cook, stirring frequently, until apples are softened and tender, about 6 to 9 minutes.

3. Put one warm waffle each on a plate, top each with yogurt and apples. Serve warm.

Nutrition:

Calories: 240 calories

Total Fat: 10.4 g

Cholesterol: 54 mg

Sodium: 226 mg

Total Carbohydrate: 33.8 g

Protein: 4.7 g

Choco Macadamia Smoothie

Preparation Time: 5 minutes Cooking Time: 5 minutes Serve: 1

Ingredients:

- 1 tbsp unsweetened cocoa powder
- 2 tbsp chia seed
- 1 tbsp coconut butter
- 1 tsp MCT oil
- 2 tbsp macadamia nuts
- 1 cup unsweetened almond milk

Directions:

- Add all ingredients into the blender and blend until smooth.
- Serve and enjoy.

Nutritional Value (Amount per Serving):

Calories 368

Fat 35.2 g

Carbohydrates 13.7 g

Sugar 1.8 g

Protein 7.5 g

Cholesterol 0 mg

Chaffle Ice Cream Bowl

Preparation Time: 5 minutes

Cooking Time: 0 minutes

Servings: 2

Ingredients:

- 4 basic chaffles
- 2 scoops keto ice cream
- 2 teaspoons sugar-free chocolate syrup

Method:

1. Arrange 2 basic chaffles in a bowl, following the contoured design of the bowl.
2. Top with the ice cream.
3. Drizzle with the syrup on top.
4. Serve.

Nutritional Value:

- Calories 181
- Total Fat 17.2g
- Saturated Fat 4.2g
- Cholesterol 26mg
- Sodium 38mg
- Total Carbohydrate 7g
- Dietary Fiber 1g
- Total Sugars 4.1g

- Protein 0.4g
- Potassium 0mg

Zucchini Chaffle

Preparation Time: 10 minutes

Cooking Time: 8 minutes

Servings: 2

Ingredients:

- 1 cup zucchini, grated
- ¼ cup mozzarella cheese, shredded
- 1 egg, beaten
- ½ cup Parmesan cheese, shredded
- 1 teaspoon dried basil
- Salt and pepper to taste

Method:

1. Preheat your waffle maker.
2. Sprinkle pinch of salt over the zucchini and mix.
3. Let sit for 2 minutes.
4. Wrap zucchini with paper towel and squeeze to get rid of water.
5. Transfer to a bowl and stir in the rest of the ingredients.
6. Pour half of the mixture into the waffle maker.
7. Close the device.
8. Cook for 4 minutes.
9. Make the second chaffle following the same steps.

Nutritional Value:

- Calories 194
- Total Fat 13 g
- Saturated Fat 7 g
- Cholesterol 115 mg
- Sodium 789 mg
- Potassium 223 mg
- Total Carbohydrate 4 g
- Dietary Fiber 1 g
- Protein 16 g
- Total Sugars 2 g

Taco Chaffle

Preparation Time: 15 minutes

Cooking Time: 20 minutes

Servings: 4

Ingredients:

- 1 tablespoon olive oil
- 1 lb. ground beef
- 1 teaspoon ground cumin
- 1 teaspoon chili powder
- ¼ teaspoon onion powder
- ½ teaspoon garlic powder
- Salt to taste
- 4 basic chaffles
- 1 cup cabbage, chopped
- 4 tablespoons salsa (sugar-free)

Method:

1. Pour the olive oil into a pan over medium heat.
2. Add the ground beef.
3. Season with the salt and spices.
4. Cook until brown and crumbly.
5. Fold the chaffle to create a "taco shell".
6. Stuff each chaffle taco with cabbage.
7. Top with the ground beef and salsa.

Nutritional Value:

- Calories 255
- Total Fat 10.9g
- Saturated Fat 3.2g
- Cholesterol 101mg
- Sodium 220mg
- Potassium 561mg
- Total Carbohydrate 3g
- Dietary Fiber 1g
- Protein 35.1g
- Total Sugars 1.3g

Chaffle Cream Cake

Preparation Time: 20 minutes

Cooking Time: 30 minutes

Servings: 8

Ingredients:

Chaffle

- 4 oz. cream cheese
- 4 eggs
- 1 tablespoon butter, melted
- 1 teaspoon vanilla extract
- ½ teaspoon cinnamon
- 1 tablespoon sweetener
- 4 tablespoons coconut flour
- 1 tablespoon almond flour
- 1 ½ teaspoons baking powder
- 1 tablespoon coconut flakes (sugar-free)
- 1 tablespoon walnuts, chopped

Frosting

- 2 oz. cream cheese
- 2 tablespoons butter
- 2 tablespoons sweetener
- ½ teaspoon vanilla

Method:

1. Combine all the chaffle ingredients except coconut flakes and walnuts in a blender.
2. Blend until smooth.
3. Plug in your waffle maker.
4. Add some of the mixture to the waffle maker.
5. Cook for 3 minutes.
6. Repeat steps until the remaining batter is used.
7. While letting the chaffles cool, make the frosting by combining all the ingredients.
8. Use a mixer to combine and turn frosting into fluffy consistency.
9. Spread the frosting on top of the chaffles.

<u>Nutritional Value:</u>

- Calories 127
- Total Fat 13.7g
- Saturated Fat 9 g
- Cholesterol 102.9mg
- Sodium 107.3mg
- Potassium 457 mg
- Total Carbohydrate 5.5g
- Dietary Fiber 1.3g
- Protein 5.3g
- Total Sugars 1.5g

Chicken Parmesan Chaffle

Preparation Time: 15 minutes

Cooking Time: 8 minutes

Servings: 2

Ingredients:

Chaffle

- 1 egg, beaten
- ¼ cup cheddar cheese, shredded
- 1/8 cup Parmesan cheese, grated
- 1 teaspoon cream cheese
- ½ cup chicken breast meat, shredded
- 1/8 teaspoon garlic powder
- 1 teaspoon Italian seasoning

Toppings

- 1 tablespoon pizza sauce (sugar-free)
- 2 provolone cheese slices

Method:

1. Plug in your waffle maker.
2. Combine all the chaffle ingredients in a bowl.
3. Mix well.
4. Add half of the mixture to the waffle maker.

5. Cook for 4 minutes.

6. Repeat with the next chaffle.

7. Spread the pizza sauce on top of each chaffle and put Provolone on top.

<u>Nutritional Value:</u>

- Calories125
- Total Fat 8.3g
- Saturated Fat 4 g
- Cholesterol 115.3mg
- Sodium 285.7mg
- Potassium 760 mg
- Total Carbohydrate 2.6g
- Dietary Fiber 0.3g
- Protein 9.4g

Chicken Chaffle

Sandwich

Preparation Time: 5 minutes

Cooking Time: 15 minutes

Servings: 2

Ingredients:

- 1 chicken breast fillet, sliced into strips
- Salt and pepper to taste
- 1 teaspoon dried rosemary
- 1 tablespoon olive oil
- 4 basic chaffles
- 2 tablespoons butter, melted
- 2 tablespoons Parmesan cheese, grated

Method:

1. Season the chicken strips with salt, pepper and rosemary.
2. Add olive oil to a pan over medium low heat.
3. Cook the chicken until brown on both sides.
4. Spread butter on top of each chaffle.
5. Sprinkle cheese on top.
6. Place the chicken on top and top with another chaffle.

Nutritional Value:

- Calories 262
- Total Fat 20g
- Saturated Fat 9.2g

- Cholesterol 77mg
- Sodium 270mg
- Potassium 125mg
- Total Carbohydrate 1g
- Dietary Fiber 0.2g
- Protein 20.2g
- Total Sugars 0g

Cornbread Chaffle

Preparation Time: 5 minutes

Cooking Time: 8 minutes

Servings: 2

Ingredients:

- 1 egg, beaten
- ½ cup cheddar cheese, shredded
- 5 slices pickled jalapeno, chopped and drained
- 1 teaspoon hot sauce
- ¼ teaspoon corn extract
- Salt to taste

Method:

1. Combine all the ingredients in a bowl while preheating your waffle maker.
2. Add half of the mixture to the device.
3. Seal and cook for 4 minutes.
4. Let cool on a plate for 2 minutes.
5. Repeat steps for the second chaffle.

Nutritional Value:

- Calories150
- Total Fat 11.8g
- Saturated Fat 7 g
- Cholesterol 121mg
- Sodium 1399.4mg
- Potassium 350 mg

- Total Carbohydrate 1.1g
- Dietary Fiber 0g
- Protein 9.6g
- Total Sugars 0.2g

Italian Sausage Chaffles

Preparation Time: 5 minutes

Cooking Time: 8 minutes

Servings: 2

Ingredients:

- 1 egg, beaten
- 1 cup cheddar cheese, shredded
- ¼ cup Parmesan cheese, grated
- 1 lb. Italian sausage, crumbled
- 2 teaspoons baking powder
- 1 cup almond flour

Method:

1. Preheat your waffle maker.
2. Mix all the ingredients in a bowl.
3. Pour half of the mixture into the waffle maker.
4. Cover and cook for 4 minutes.
5. Transfer to a plate.
6. Let cool to make it crispy.
7. Do the same steps to make the next chaffle.

Nutritional Value:

- Calories 332
- Total Fat 27.1g
- Saturated Fat 10.2g

- Cholesterol 98mg
- Sodium 634mg
- Total Carbohydrate 1.9g
- Dietary Fiber 0.5g
- Total Sugars 0.1g
- Protein 19.6g
- Potassium 359mg

Cheese Garlic

Chaffle

Preparation Time: 10 minutes

Cooking Time: 8 minutes

Servings: 2

Ingredients:

Chaffle

- 1 egg
- 1 teaspoon cream cheese
- ½ cup mozzarella cheese, shredded
- ½ teaspoon garlic powder
- 1 teaspoon Italian seasoning

Topping

- 1 tablespoon butter
- ½ teaspoon garlic powder
- ½ teaspoon Italian seasoning
- 2 tablespoon mozzarella cheese, shredded

Method:

1. Plug in your waffle maker to preheat.
2. Preheat your oven to 350 degrees F.
3. In a bowl, combine all the chaffle ingredients.
4. Cook in the waffle maker for 4 minutes per chaffle.
5. Transfer to a baking pan.

6. Spread butter on top of each chaffle.

7. Sprinkle garlic powder and Italian seasoning on top.

8. Top with mozzarella cheese.

9. Bake until the cheese has melted.

Nutritional Value:

- Calories141
- Total Fat 13 g
- Saturated Fat 8 g
- Cholesterol 115.8 mg
- Sodium 255.8 mg
- Potassium 350 mg
- Total Carbohydrate 2.6g
- Dietary Fiber 0.7g

Energy Booster Breakfast Smoothie

Preparation Time: 5 minutes Cooking Time: 5 minutes
Serve: 1

Ingredients:

- 1 cup unsweetened almond milk
- 1/2 cup ice
- 1 1/2 tsp maca powder
- 1 tbsp almond butter
- 1 tbsp MCT oil

Directions:

1. Add all ingredients into the blender and blend until smooth.
2. Serve and enjoy.

Nutritional Value (Amount per Serving):

Calories 248

Fat 26.5 g

Carbohydrates 4.5 g

Sugar 1.2 g

Protein 4.9 g

Cholesterol 0 mg

Blackberry

Smoothie

Preparation Time: 5 minutes Cooking Time: 5
minutes

Serve: 2

Ingredients:

- 1 cup unsweetened almond milk
- 1/2 cup ice
- 1/2 tsp vanilla
- 1 tsp erythritol
- 2 oz cream cheese, softened
- 4 tbsp heavy whipping cream
- 2 oz fresh blackberries

Directions:

1. Add all ingredients into the blender and blend until smooth.
2. Serve and enjoy.

Nutritional Value (Amount per Serving):

Calories 238

Fat 22.9 g

Carbohydrates 5.9 g

Sugar 4.1 g

Protein 3.7 g

Cholesterol 72 mg

SEAFOOD & FISH
RECIPES

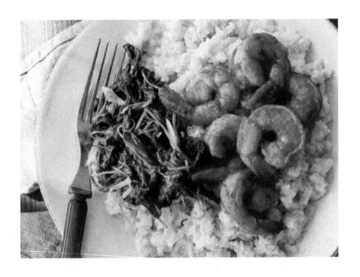

Buttery Shrimp

Preparation Time: 5 minutes Cooking Time: 15
minutes

Serve: 4

Ingredients:

- 1 1/2 lbs shrimp
- 1 tbsp Italian seasoning
- 1 lemon, sliced
- 1 stick butter, melted

Directions:

1. Add all ingredients into the large mixing bowl and
   toss well.
2. Transfer shrimp mixture on baking tray.
3. Bake at 350 F for 15 minutes.
4. Serve and enjoy.

Nutritional Value (Amount per Serving):

Calories 415

Fat 26 g

Carbohydrates 3 g

Sugar 0.3 g

Protein 39 g

Cholesterol 421 mg

MEATLESS
MEALS

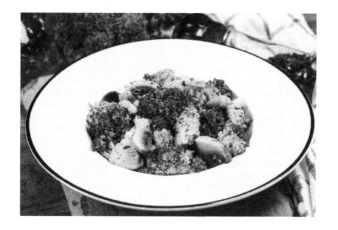

Mexican

Cauliflower Rice

Preparation Time: 10 minutes Cooking Time: 10 minutes Serve: 3

Ingredients:

- 1 large cauliflower head, cut into florets
- 2 garlic cloves, minced
- 1 onion, diced
- 1 tbsp olive oil
- 1/4 cup vegetable broth
- 3 tbsp tomato paste
- 1/2 tsp cumin
- 1 tsp salt

Directions:

1. Add cauliflower in food processor and process until it looks like rice.
2. Heat oil in a pan over medium heat.
3. Add onion and garlic and sauté for 3 minutes.
4. Add cauliflower rice, cumin, and salt and stir well.
5. Add broth and tomato paste and stir until well combined.
6. Serve and enjoy.

Nutritional Value (Amount per Serving):

Calories 90

Fat 5 g

Carbohydrates 10 g

Sugar 4 g

Protein 3 g

Cholesterol 0 mg

Balsamic Zucchini
Noodles

Preparation Time: 10 minutes Cooking Time: 15 minutes Serve: 4

Ingredients:

- 4 zucchinis, spiralized using a slicer
- 1 1/2 tbsp balsamic vinegar
- 1/4 cup fresh basil leaves, chopped
- 4 mozzarella balls, quartered
- 1 1/2 cups cherry tomatoes, halved
- 2 tbsp olive oil
- Pepper
- Salt

Directions:

1. Add zucchini noodles in a bowl and season with pepper and salt. Set aside for 10 minutes.
2. Add mozzarella, tomatoes, and basil and toss well.
3. Drizzle with oil and balsamic vinegar.
4. Serve and enjoy.

Nutritional Value (Amount per Serving):

Calories 222

Fat 15 g

Carbohydrates 10 g

Sugar 5.8 g

Protein 9.5 g

Cholesterol 13 mg

SOUPS, STEWS
& SALADS

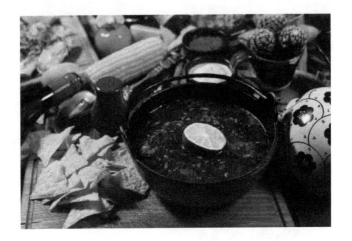

Avocado Soup

Preparation Time: 10 minutes Cooking Time: 10 minutes

Serve: 6

Ingredients:

- 2 avocados, peel and pitted
- 1 cup heavy cream
- 2 tbsp dry sherry
- 2 cups vegetable broth
- ½ tsp fresh lemon juice
- Pepper
- Salt

Directions:

1. Add avocado, lemon juice, sherry, and broth to the blender and blend until smooth.
2. Pour blended mixture into a bowl and stir in cream.
3. Season with pepper and salt.
4. Serve and enjoy.

Nutritional Value (Amount per Serving):

Calories 102

Fat 9.5 g

Carbohydrates 1.9 g

Sugar 0.3 g

Protein 2.4 g

Cholesterol 27 m

BRUNCH & DINNER

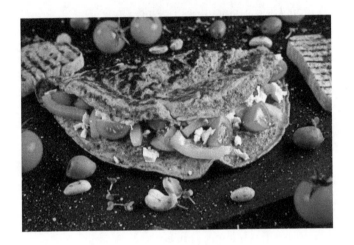

Olive Cheese Omelet

Preparation Time: 10 minutes Cooking Time: 5 minutes

Serve: 4

Ingredients:

- 4 large eggs
- 2 oz cheese
- 12 olives, pitted
- 2 tbsp butter
- 2 tbsp olive oil
- 1 tsp herb de Provence
- 1/2 tsp salt

Directions:

1. Add all ingredients except butter in a bowl whisk well until frothy.
2. Melt butter in a pan over medium heat.
3. Pour egg mixture onto hot pan and spread evenly.
4. Cover and cook for 3 minutes.
5. Turn omelet to other side and cook for 2 minutes more.
6. Serve and enjoy.

Nutritional Value (Amount per Serving):

Calories 250

Fat 23 g

Carbohydrates 2 g

Sugar 1 g

Protein 10 g

Cholesterol 216 mg

DESSERTS & DRINKS

Choco Frosty

Preparation Time: 5 minutes Cooking Time: 5 minutes

Serve: 4

Ingredients:

- 1 tsp vanilla
- 8 drops liquid stevia
- 2 tbsp unsweetened cocoa powder
- 1 tbsp almond butter
- 1 cup heavy cream

Directions:

1. Add all ingredients into the mixing bowl and beat with immersion blender
   until soft peaks form.
2. Place in refrigerator for 30 minutes.
3. Add frosty mixture into the piping bag and pipe in serving glasses.
4. Serve and enjoy.

Nutritional Value (Amount per Serving):

Calories 240

Fat 25 g

Carbohydrates 4 g

Sugar 3 g

Protein 3 g

Cholesterol 43 mg

BREAKFAST RECIPES

Iced Matcha Latte

Serves: 1

Prep Time: 10 mins

Ingredients

- 1 tablespoon coconut oil
- 1 cup unsweetened cashew milk
- 1 teaspoon matcha powder
- 2 ice cubes
- 1/8 teaspoon vanilla bean

Directions

1. Mix together all the ingredients in a blender and blend until smooth.
2. Pour into a glass to serve.

Nutrition Amount per serving

Calories 161

Total Fat 16g 21% Saturated Fat 12g 60%

Cholesterol 3mg 1%

Sodium 166mg   7%

Total Carbohydrate 2.9g 1% Dietary Fiber 2g 7%

Total Sugars 1.4g Protein 2.4g

Browned Butter

Pumpkin Latte

Serves: 2

Prep Time: 10 mins

Ingredients

- 2 shots espresso

- 2 tablespoons butter

- 2 scoops Stevia

- 2 cups hot almond milk

- 4 tablespoons pumpkin puree

Directions

1. Heat butter on low heat in a small pan and allow to lightly brown.

2. Brew two shots of espresso and stir in the Stevia.

3. Add browned butter along with pumpkin puree and hot almond milk.

4. Blend for about 10 seconds on high and pour into 2 cups to serve.

Nutrition Amount per serving

Calories 227

Total Fat 22.6g 29% Saturated Fat 18.3g 92%

Cholesterol 31mg 10%

Sodium 93mg 4%

Total Carbohydrate 4.5g 2% Dietary Fiber 0.9g 3%

Total Sugars 1g, Protein 1.5g

APPETIZERS AND DESSERTS

Caprese Snack

Serves: 4

Prep Time: 5 mins

Ingredients

- 8 oz. mozzarella, mini cheese balls
- 8 oz. cherry tomatoes
- 2 tablespoons green pesto
- Salt and black pepper, to taste
- 1 tablespoon garlic powder

Directions

1. Slice the mozzarella balls and tomatoes in half.
2. Stir in the green pesto and season with garlic powder, salt and pepper to serve.

Nutrition Amount per serving

Calories 407

Total Fat 34.5g 44% Saturated Fat 7.4g 37%

Cholesterol 30mg 10%

Sodium 343mg 15%

Total Carbohydrate 6.3g 2% Dietary Fiber 0.9g 3%

Total Sugars 2g Protein 19.4g

PORK, BEEF &
LAMB RECIPES

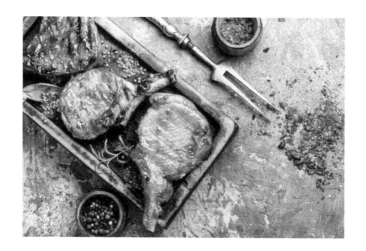

Spinach Pork Roll Ups

Serves: 8

Prep Time: 15 mins

Ingredients

- 2 teaspoons honey mustard

- 8 thin slices bacon, smoked

- 1 cup Monterey Jack cheese, cut lengthwise into quarters

- 1 cup fresh baby spinach leaves

- ½ medium red bell pepper, seeded and cut into thin strips

Directions

1. Spread the honey mustard over bacon slices.
2. Divide spinach leaves among 8 plates and place bacon slices on it.
3. Top with red bell pepper and cheese to serve.

Nutrition Amount per serving

Calories 161

Total Fat 12.3g 16%

Saturated Fat 5.3g 27%

Cholesterol 33mg 11%

Sodium 524mg 23%

Total Carbohydrate 1.6g 1%

Dietary Fiber 0.2g 1%

Total Sugars 0.7g

Protein 10.7g

Pork with Butternut Squash Stew

Serves: 4

Prep Time: 40 mins

Ingredients

- ½ pound butternut squash, peeled and cubed

- 1 pound lean pork

- 2 tablespoons butter

- Salt and black pepper, to taste

- 1 cup beef stock

Directions

1. Put the butter and lean pork in a skillet and cook for about 5 minutes.
2. Add butternut squash, beef stock and season with salt and black pepper.
3. Cover with lid and cook for about 25 minutes on medium low heat.
4. Dish out to a bowl and serve hot.

Nutrition Amount per serving

Calories 319

Total Fat 17.1g 22% Satu-

rated Fat 7.9g 39% Choles-

terol 105mg 35%

Sodium 311mg 14%

Total Carbohydrate 6.7g 2%

Dietary Fiber 1.1g 4%

Total Sugars 1.3g

Protein 33.7g

Keto Taco Casserole

Serves: 8

Prep Time: 55 mins

Ingredients

- 2 pounds ground beef

- 1 tablespoon extra-virgin olive oil

- Taco seasoning mix, kosher salt and black pepper

- 2 cups Mexican cheese, shredded

- 6 large eggs, lightly beaten

Directions

1. Preheat the oven to 3600F and grease a 2 quart baking dish.
2. Heat oil over medium heat in a large skillet and add ground beef.
3. Season with taco seasoning mix, kosher salt and black pepper.
4. Cook for about 5 minutes on each side and dish out to let cool slightly.
5. Whisk together eggs in the beef mixture and transfer the mixture to the baking dish.
6. Top with Mexican cheese and bake for about 25 minutes until set.
7. Remove from the oven and serve warm.

Nutrition Amount per serving

Calories 382

Total Fat 21.6g 28% Satu-
rated Fat 9.1g 45% Cho-
lesterol 266mg 89%

Sodium 363mg 16%

Total Carbohydrate 1.7g 1%

Dietary Fiber 0g 0%

Total Sugars 0.4g

Protein 45.3g

Hamburger Patties

Serves: 6

Prep Time: 30 mins

Ingredients

- 1 egg
- 25 oz. ground beef
- 3 oz. feta cheese, crumbled
- 2 oz. butter, for frying
- Salt and black pepper, to taste

Directions

1. Mix together egg, ground beef, feta cheese, salt and black pepper in a bowl.
2. Combine well and form equal sized patties.
3. Heat butter in a pan and add patties.
4. Cook on medium low heat for about 3 minutes per side.
5. Dish out and serve warm.

Nutrition Amount per serving

Calories 335

Total Fat 18.8g 24% Saturated Fat 10g 50%

Cholesterol 166mg 55%

Sodium 301mg   13%

Total Carbohydrate 0.7g 0% Dietary Fiber 0g 0%

Total Sugars 0.7g Protein 38.8g

Beef Roast

Serves: 6

Prep Time: 55 mins

Ingredients

- 2 pounds beef
- Salt and black pepper, to taste
- 1 cup onion soup
- 2 teaspoons lemon juice
- 1 cups beef broth

Directions

1. Put the beef in a pressure cooker and stir in the beef broth, lemon juice, onion soup, salt and black pepper.
2. Lock the lid and cook at High Pressure for about 40 minutes.
3. Naturally release the pressure and dish out on a platter to serve.

Nutrition Amount per serving

Calories 307

Total Fat 10.2g 13% Saturated Fat 3.7g 19%

Cholesterol 135mg 45%

Sodium 580mg 25%

Total Carbohydrate 2.9g 1% Dietary Fiber 0.3g 1%

Total Sugars 1.3g Protein 47.9g

Stuffed Pork Chops

Serves: 6

Prep Time: 40 mins

Ingredients

- 4 garlic cloves, minced

- 2 pounds cut boneless pork chops

- 1½ teaspoons salt

- 8 oz. provolone cheese

- 2 cups baby spinach

Directions

1. Preheat the oven to 3500F and grease a baking sheet
2. Mix garlic with salt and rub on one side of the pork chops.
3. Place half of the pork chops garlic side down on a baking sheet and top with spinach and provolone cheese.
4. Top with rest of the pork chops garlic side up and place in the oven.
5. Bake for about 30 minutes and dish out to serve hot

SEAFOOD RECIPES

Garlic Shrimp with Goat Cheese

Serves: 4

Prep Time: 30 mins

Ingredients

- 4 tablespoons herbed butter
- Salt and black pepper, to taste
- 1 pound large raw shrimp
- 4 ounces goat cheese
- 4 garlic cloves, chopped

Directions

1. Preheat the oven to 3750F and grease a baking dish.
2. Mix together herbed butter, garlic, raw shrimp, salt and black pepper in a bowl.
3. Put the marinated shrimp on the baking dish and top with the shredded cheese.
4. Place in the oven and bake for about 25 minutes.
5. Take the shrimp out and serve hot.

Nutrition Amount per serving

Calories 294

Total Fat 15g 19% Saturated Fat 8.9g 44% Cholesterol

266mg 89%

Sodium 392mg 17%

Total Carbohydrate 2.1g 1% Dietary Fiber 0.1g 0%

Total Sugars 0.8g Protein 35.8g

Browned Butter

Cauliflower Mash

Serves: 4

Prep Time: 35 mins

Ingredients

- 1 yellow onion, finely chopped
- ¾ cup heavy whipping cream
- 1½ pounds cauliflower, shredded
- Sea salt and black pepper, to taste
- 3½ oz. butter

Directions

1. Heat 2 tablespoons butter in a skillet on medium heat and add onions.
2. Sauté for about 3 minutes and dish out to a bowl.
3. Mix together cauliflower, heavy whipping cream, sea salt and black pepper in the same skillet.
4. Cover with lid and cook on medium low heat for about 15 minutes.
5. Season with salt and black pepper and stir in sautéed onions.
6. Dish out to a bowl and heat the rest of the butter in the

55

skillet.

7. Cook until the butter is brown and nutty and serve with cauliflower mash.

Nutrition Amount per serving

Calories 309

Total Fat 28.7g 37% Saturated Fat 18g 90%

Cholesterol 84mg 28%

Sodium 204mg 9%

Total Carbohydrate 12.2g 4% Dietary Fiber 4.8g 17%

Total Sugars 5.3g Protein 4.3g

CHICKEN AND POULTRY RECIPES

Turkey with Cream Cheese Sauce

Serves: 4

Prep Time: 30 mins

Ingredients

- 20 oz. turkey breast
- 2 tablespoons butter
- 2 cups heavy whipping cream
- Salt and black pepper, to taste
- 7 oz. cream cheese

Directions

1. Season the turkey generously with salt and black pepper.
2. Heat butter in a skillet over medium heat and cook turkey for about 5 minutes on each side.
3. Stir in the heavy whipping cream and cream cheese.
4. Cover the skillet and cook for about 15 minutes on medium low heat.
5. Dish out to serve hot.

Nutrition Amount per serving

Calories 386

Total Fat 31.7g 41% Saturated Fat 19.2g 96%

Cholesterol 142mg 47%

Sodium 1100mg 48% Total Carbohydrate 6g 2%

Dietary Fiber 0.5g 2% Total Sugars 3.4g

Protein 19.5g

BREAKFAST RECIPES

Almond Hemp Heart Porridge

Total Time: 10 minutes

Serves: 2

Ingredients:

- ¼ cup almond flour
- ½ tsp cinnamon
- ¾ tsp vanilla extract
- 5 drops stevia
- 1 tbsp chia seeds
- 2 tbsp ground flax seed
- ½ cup hemp hearts
- 1 cup unsweetened coconut milk

Directions:

1. Add all ingredients except almond flour to a saucepan. Stir to combine.
2. Heat over medium heat until just starts to lightly boil.
3. Once start bubbling then stir well and cook for 1 minute more.

59

4. Remove from heat and stir in almond flour.

5. Serve immediately and enjoy.

Nutritional Value (Amount per Serving): Calories 329; Fat 24.4 g; Carbohydrates 9.2 g; Sugar 1.8 g; Protein 16.2 g; Cholesterol 0 mg;

Flax Almond

Muffins

Total Time: 45 minutes Serves: 6

Ingredients:

- 1 tsp cinnamon
- 2 tbsp coconut flour
- 20 drops liquid stevia
- 1/4 cup water
- 1/4 tsp vanilla extract
- 1/4 tsp baking soda
- 1/2 tsp baking powder
- 1/4 cup almond flour
- 1/2 cup ground flax
- 2 tbsp ground chia

Directions:

Preheat the oven to 350 F/ 176 C.

1. Spray muffin tray with cooking spray and set aside.
2. In a small bowl, add 6 tablespoons of water and ground chia. Mix well and set aside.
3. In a mixing bowl, add ground flax, baking soda, baking powder, cinnamon, coconut flour, and almond flour and mix well.
4. Add chia seed mixture, vanilla, water, and liquid stevia and stir well to combine.

5. Pour mixture into the prepared muffin tray and bake in preheated oven for 35 minutes.

6. Serve and enjoy.

Nutritional Value (Amount per Serving): Calories 92; Fat 6.3 g; Carbohydrates 6.9 g;

Sugar 0.4 g; Protein 3.7 g; Cholesterol 0 mg;

LUNCH RECIPES

Lemon Zucchini Noodles

Total Time: 15 minutes Serves: 4

Ingredients:

- 4 small zucchini, spiralized into noodles
- 2 garlic cloves
- 2 cups fresh basil leaves
- 2 tsp lemon juice
- 1/3 cup olive oil
- Pepper
- Salt

Directions:

1. Add garlic, basil, olive oil, and lemon juice into the blender and blend well. Season with pepper and salt.
2. In a large bowl, combine together pesto and zucchini noodles.
3. Stir well and serve.

Nutritional Value (Amount per Serving): Calories 169; Fat 17.1 g; Carbohydrates 4.8 g; Sugar 2.2 g; Protein 1.9 g; Cholesterol 0 mg;

Mexican Cauliflower Rice

Total Time: 25 minutes Serves: 4

Ingredients:

- 1 medium cauliflower head, cut into florets
- ½ cup tomato sauce
- ¼ tsp black pepper
- 1 tsp chili powder
- 2 garlic cloves, minced
- ½ medium onion, diced
- 1 tbsp coconut oil
- ½ tsp sea sal

Directions:

1. Add cauliflower florets into the food processor and process until it looks like rice.
2. Heat oil in a pan over medium-high heat.
3. Add onion to the pan and sauté for 5 minutes or until softened.
4. Add garlic and cook for 1 minute.
5. Add cauliflower rice, chili powder, pepper, and salt. Stir well.
6. Add tomato sauce and cook for 5 minutes.
7. Stir well and serve warm.

Nutritional Value (Amount per Serving): Calories 83; Fat 3.7g; Carbohydrates 11.5 g; Sugar 5.4 g; Protein 3.6 g; Cholesterol 0 mg;

DINNER RECIPES

Lemon Garlic

Mushrooms

Total Time: 25 minutes Serves: 4

Ingredients:

- 3 oz enoki mushrooms
- 1 tbsp olive oil
- 1 tsp lemon zest, chopped
- 2 tbsp lemon juice
- 3 garlic cloves, sliced
- 6 oyster mushrooms, halved
- 5 oz cremini mushrooms, sliced
- 1/2 red chili, sliced
- 1/2 onion, sliced
- 1 tsp sea salt

Directions:

1. Heat olive oil in a pan over high heat.
2. Add shallots, enoki mushrooms, oyster mushrooms, cremini mushrooms, and chili.
3. Stir well and cook over medium-high heat for 10

minutes.

4. Add lemon zest and stir well. Season with lemon juice and salt and cook for 3-4 minutes.

5. Serve and enjoy.

Nutritional Value (Amount per Serving): Calories 87; Fat 5.6 g; Carbohydrates 7.5 g;

Sugar 1.8 g; Protein 3 g; Cholesterol 8 mg;

Tomato Asparagus Salad

Total Time: 20 minutes Serves: 4

Ingredients:

- 1/2 lb asparagus, trimmed and cut into pieces
- 8 oz cherry tomatoes, halved
- For dressing:
- 1/4 tsp garlic and herb seasoning blend
- 1 tbsp vinegar
- 1 tbsp shallot, minced
- 1 garlic clove, minced
- 1 tbsp water
- 2 tbsp olive oil

Directions:

1. Add 1 tablespoon of water and asparagus in a heatproof bowl and cover with cling film and microwave for 2 minutes.
2. Remove asparagus from bowl and place into ice water until cool.
3. Add asparagus and tomatoes into a medium bowl.
4. In a small bowl, mix together all remaining ingredients and pour over vegetables.
5. Toss vegetables well and serve.

Nutritional Value (Amount per Serving): Calories 85; Fat 7.2 g; Carbohydrates 5.1 g;

Sugar 2.6 g; Protein 1.9 g; Cholesterol 0 mg;

DESSERT RECIPES

Lemon Mousse

Total Time: 10 minutes Serves: 2

Ingredients:

- 14 oz coconut milk
- 12 drops liquid stevia
- 1/2 tsp lemon extract
- 1/4 tsp turmeric

Directions:

1. Place coconut milk can in the refrigerator for overnight. Scoop out thick cream into a mixing bowl.
2. Add remaining ingredients to the bowl and whip using a hand mixer until smooth.
3. Transfer mousse mixture to a zip-lock bag and pipe into small serving glasses. Place in refrigerator.
4. Serve chilled and enjoy.

Nutritional Value (Amount per Serving): Calories 444; Fat 45.7 g; Carbohydrates 10 g; Sugar 6 g; Protein 4.4 g; Cholesterol 0 mg;

BREAKFAST RECIPES

Almond Butter

Shake

Get your morning started right with this fantastic boost in energy that takes just 5 minutes to make.

Total Prep & Cooking Time: 5 minutes Level: Beginner

Makes: 1 Shake

Protein: 19 grams Net Carbs: 6 grams Fat:

27 grams

Sugar: 0 grams

Calories: 326

What you need:

- 1 1/2 cups almond milk, unsweetened
- 2 tbs almond butter
- 1/2 tbs ground cinnamon
- 2 tbs flax meal
- 1/8 tsp almond extract, sugar-free
- 15 drops liquid Stevia
- 1/8 tsp salt
- 6 ice cubes

Steps:

Using a blender, combine all the listed ingredients and pulse for approximately 45 seconds.

Serve immediately and enjoy!

LUNCH RECIPES

Egg Salad

Whip this egg salad up in no time and enjoy the fantastic boost in energy from this fat bomb.

Total Prep & Cooking Time: 15 minutes Level: Beginner

Makes: 2 Helpings

Protein: 6 grams Net Carbs: 1 gram Fat:

28 grams

Sugar: 1 gram

Calories: 260

What you need:

- 3 tbs mayonnaise, sugar-free
- 1/4 cup celery, chopped
- 2 large eggs, hardboiled and yolks separated.
- 1/2 tsp mustard
- 3 tbs red bell pepper, chopped
- 1/4 tsp salt
- 3 tbs broccoli, riced
- 1/4 tsp pepper
- 2 tbs mushroom, chopped
- 1/4 tsp paprika
- 4 cups cold water

Steps:

1. Fill a saucepan with the eggs and 2 cups of the cold water.

2. When the water begins to boil, set a timer for 7 minutes.

3. After the time has passed, drain the water and empty the remaining 2 cups of cold water over the eggs.

4. Once they can be handled, peel the eggs and remove the yolks. Chop the egg whites and leave to the side.

5. In a large dish, blend the mayonnaise, mustard, salt and egg yolks.

6. Combine the chopped celery, bell pepper, broccoli, and mushroom.

7. Finally, integrate the egg whites, pepper and paprika until combined fully.

SNACK RECIPES

Bacon Wrapped Avocado

This quick fried snack is going to have you filling up on the nutrients and fats that your
body craves.

Total Prep & Cooking Time: 30 minutes Level: Beginner

Makes: 3 Helpings (2 wraps per serving) Protein: 15 grams

Net Carbs: 1.8 grams Fat: 21 grams

Sugar: 0 grams

Calories: 139

What you need:

- 1 avocado, peeled and pitted
- 6 strips bacon
- 1 tbs butter

Steps:

1. Slice the avocado into 6 individual wedges.
2. Wrap one slice of bacon around the avocado wedge and repeat for all pieces.
3. Soften the butter in a non-stick skillet and transfer the wedges to the hot butter with the end of the bacon on the

base of the pan. This will prevent the bacon from coming apart from the wedge.

4. Cook for approximately 3 minutes on each side, and move to a paper towel covered plate.

5. Serve while still hot and enjoy!

Baking Tip:

Do not use an avocado that is mushy or overripe as it will crumble while wrapping with the bacon.

Variation Tip:

You can also substitute asparagus instead of the avocado.

DINNER
RECIPES

Chicken Kebab

When you sink your teeth into this flavorful shawarma, you will not be missing the bread that used to come with it.

Total Prep & Cooking Time: 45 minutes plus 2 hours to marinate

Level: Beginner Makes: 4 Helpings

Protein: 35 grams Net Carbs: 1 gram Fat: 16

grams

Sugar: 0 grams

Calories: 274

What you need:

For the chicken:

- 21 oz. boneless chicken breast or thighs
- 2/3 tsp ground coriander
- 6 tsp olive oil
- 2/3 tsp ground cumin
- 1/3 tsp ground cayenne pepper
- 2/3 tsp ground cardamom
- 1/3 tsp garlic powder
- 2/3 tsp ground turmeric
- 1/3 tsp onion powder
- 2 tsp paprika powder 77
- 1 tsp salt

- 4 tsp lemon juice
- 1/8 tsp pepper

For the tahini sauce:
- 4 tsp olive oil
- 2 tbs water
- 1/3 tsp salt
- 4 tsp tahini paste
- 2 tsp lemon juice
- 1 clove garlic, minced

Steps:

1. With a rubber scraper, blend the coriander, olive oil, cumin, cayenne pepper, cardamom, garlic powder, turmeric, onion powder, paprika powder, salt, lemon juice and pepper in a big lidded tub.

2. Place the chicken inside and arrange, so they are covered completely by the liquid.

3. Marinate for at least 2 hours, if not overnight.

4. Preheat your grill to heat at 500° Fahrenheit.

5. Take away the chicken from the marinade and grill over the flames for approximately 4 minutes before flipping to the other side.

6. Grill until browned on both sides and use a meat thermometer to ensure it is a uniform 160° Fahrenheit.

7. Take away the chicken to a plate and cool for about 10

minutes.

8. In a small dish, blend the olive oil, water, salt, tahini paste, lemon, and minced garlic until a smooth consistency.

9. Slice the chicken and serve with the sauce and enjoy!

Baking Tips:

1. If you do not own a grill, you can fry this meal on the stove. Once the chicken is marinated, dissolve a tablespoon of butter or coconut oil in a non-stick skillet. Fry the chicken on each side for approximately 4 minutes.

2. Baking the chicken is another option. Adjust the temperature of the stove to 400° Fahrenheit and roast for approximately 20 minutes.

Variation Tip:

1. If you like a kick to your chicken, you can add more cayenne pepper to your preferred taste.

UNUSUAL DELICIOUS MEAL RECIPES

You have made it to the bonus chapter where there is a unique collection of recipes, as most are exotic and from overseas. Some have a few more steps, but they are still going to be easy enough for anyone to bring to their dinner table tonight. Enjoy experimenting with something new!

Blackberry Clafoutis Tarts

This rendition of the traditional dessert from France is very creamy and low carb to boot.

Total Prep & Cooking Time: 1 hour 30 minutes

Level: Beginner Makes: 4 Tarts

Protein: 3 grams

Net Carbs: 2.4 grams Fat: 15 grams

Sugar: 1 gram

Calories: 201

What you need:

For the crust:

- 1/4 cup coconut flour
- 2 tbs coconut oil, melted
- 2 tbs almond butter, smooth
- 1/4 tsp Swerve sweetener, confectioner
- 2 1/2 cups pecan pieces, raw
- 1/8 tsp salt

For the filling:

- 1 large egg
- 8 oz. blackberries
- 1/8 cup almond flour, blanched
- 2 oz. almond milk, unsweetened
- 3 tsp Stevia sweetener, granulated
- 1/8 tsp salt
- 3 oz. coconut milk, canned
- 1 tsp vanilla extract, sugar-free

Steps:

1. Set the stove to heat at 350° Fahrenheit. You will need to set aside four   4 3/4-inch tart pans.
2. To create the tart crusts, blend the coconut flour, Swerve, pecan pieces, salt, coconut oil, almond butter in a food blender for approximately 2 minutes until crumbly.
81
3. Scrape down the bowl with a rubber scraper and pulse

for an additional 30 seconds.

4. Portion the batter in 4 equal sections and distribute to the tart pans. Press the crust evenly by starting with the sides with the middle being pressed last. Refrigerate to set for half an hour.

5. Remove the crusts from the fridge and place a quarter cup of blackberries in each tart pan.

6. Using the food blender, whip the Stevia, vanilla extract, egg, salt, coconut milk and almond milk for approximately half a minute.

7. Empty the contents evenly over the blackberries.

8. Heat the tarts for about half an hour and remove to the counter.

9. Wait approximately 10 minutes for serving warm. Enjoy!

KETO DESSERTS RECIPES

Flavors Pumpkin Bars

Serves: 18

Preparation time: 10 minutes Cooking time: 10 minutes

Ingredients:

- 1 tbsp coconut flour
- ½ tsp cinnamon
- 2 tsp pumpkin pie spice
- 1 tsp liquid stevia
- ½ cup erythritol
- 15 oz can pumpkin puree
- 15 oz can unsweetened coconut milk
- 16 oz cocoa butter

Directions:

1. Line baking dish with parchment paper and set aside.
2. Melt cocoa butter in a small saucepan over low heat.
3. Add pumpkin puree and coconut milk and stir well.
4. Add remaining ingredients and whisk well.

5. Stir the mixture continuously until mixture thickens.

6. Once the mixture thickens then pour it into prepared baking dish and place in the refrigerator for 2 hours.

7. Slice and serve.

Per Serving: Net Carbs: 5.8g; Calories: 282; Total Fat: 28.1g; Saturated Fat: 17.1g

Protein: 1.3g; Carbs: 9.5g; Fiber: 3.7g; Sugar: 4g; Fat 89% / Protein 2% / Carbs 9%

Saffron Coconut Bars

Serves: 15

Preparation time: 10 minutes Cooking time: 15 minutes

Ingredients:

- 1 3/4 cups unsweetened shredded coconut
- 8 saffron threads
- 1 1/3 cups unsweetened coconut milk
- 1 tsp cardamom powder
- 1/4 cup Swerve
- oz ghee

Directions:

1. Spray a square baking dish with cooking spray and set aside.
2. In a bowl, mix together coconut milk and shredded coconut and set aside for half an hour.
3. Add sweetener and saffron and mix well to combine.
4. Melt ghee in a pan over medium heat.
5. Add coconut mixture to the pan and cook for 5-7 minutes.
6. Add cardamom powder and cook for 3-5 minutes more.
7. Transfer coconut mixture into the prepared baking

dish and spread evenly.

8. Place in refrigerator for 1-2 hours.

9. Slice and serve.

Per Serving: Net Carbs: 1.7g; Calories: 191 Total Fat: 19.2g; Saturated Fat: 15.1g

Protein: 1.5g; Carbs: 4.1g; Fiber: 2.4g; Sugar: 1.6g; Fat 91% / Protein 5% / Carbs 4%

CAKE

Flourless Chocó

Cake

Serves: 8

Preparation time: 10 minutes Cooking time: 45

minutes

Ingredients:

- 7 oz unsweetened dark chocolate, chopped
- ¼ cup Swerve
- 4 eggs, separated
- oz cream
- oz butter, cubed

Directions:

1. Grease 8-inch cake pan with butter and set aside.
2. Add butter and chocolate in

microwave safe bowl and microwave until melted. Stir well.

3. Add sweetener and cream and mix well.
4. Add egg yolks one by one and mix until combined.
5. In another bowl, beat egg whites until stiff peaks form.
6. Gently fold egg whites into the chocolate mixture.
7. Pour batter in the prepared cake pan and bake at 325 F/ 162 C
   for 45 minutes.
8. Slice and serve.

Per Serving: Net Carbs: 5.1g; Calories: 318; Total Fat: 28.2g; Saturated Fat: 17g

Protein: 6.6g; Carbs: 8.4g; Fiber: 3.3g; Sugar: 1.2g; Fat 82% / Protein 10% / Carbs 8%

Gooey Chocolate Cake

Serves: 8

Preparation time: 10 minutes Cooking time: 20 minutes

Ingredients:

- 2 eggs
- 1/4 cup unsweetened cocoa powder
- 1/2 cup almond flour
- 1/2 cup butter, melted
- 1 tsp vanilla
- 3/4 cup Swerve
- Pinch of salt

Directions:

1. Preheat the oven to 350 F/ 180 C.
2. Spray 8-inch spring-form cake pan with cooking spray. Set aside.
3. In a bowl, sift together almond flour, cocoa powder, and salt. Mix well and set aside.
4. In another bowl, whisk eggs, vanilla extract, and sweetener until creamy.
5. Slowly fold the almond flour mixture into the egg mixture and stir well to combine.
6. Add melted butter and stir well.
7. Pour cake batter into the prepared pan and bake for 20

minutes.

8. Remove from oven and allow to cool completely.

9. Slice and serve.

Per Serving: Net Carbs: 1.7g; Calories: 166; Total Fat: 16.5g; Saturated Fat: 8.1g

Protein: 3.5 g; Carbs: 3.3g; Fiber: 1.6g; Sugar: 0.5g; Fat 88% / Protein 8% / Carbs 4%

CANDY: BEGINNER

Strawberry Candy

Serves: 12

Preparation time: 10 minutes Cooking time: 10 minutes

Ingredients:

- 3 fresh strawberries
- 1/2 cup butter, softened
- 8 oz cream cheese, softened
- 1/2 tsp vanilla
- 3/4 cup Swerve

Directions:

1. Add all ingredients into the food processor and process until smooth.
2. Pour mixture into the silicone candy mold and place in the refrigerator for 2 hours or until candy is hardened.
3. Serve and enjoy.

Per Serving: Net Carbs: 0.8g; Calories: 136 Total Fat: 14.3g; Saturated Fat: 9g

Protein: 1.5g; Carbs: 0.9g; Fiber: 0.1g; Sugar: 0.2g; Fat 94% / Protein 4% / Carbs 2%

Blackberry Candy

Serves: 8

Preparation time: 5 minutes Cooking time: 5 minutes

Ingredients:

- 1/2 cup fresh blackberries
- 1/4 cup cashew butter
- 1 tbsp fresh lemon juice
- 1/2 cup coconut oil
- 1/2 cup unsweetened coconut milk

Directions:

1. Heat cashew butter, coconut oil, and coconut milk in a pan over medium- low heat, until just warm.
2. Transfer cashew butter mixture to the blender along with remaining ingredients and blend until smooth.
3. Pour mixture into the silicone candy mold and refrigerate until set.
4. Serve and enjoy.

Per Serving: Net Carbs: 2.9g; Calories: 203; Total Fat: 21.2g; Saturated Fat: 15.8g

Protein: 1.9g; Carbs: 3.9g; Fiber: 1g; Sugar: 1g; Fat 92% / Protein 3% / Carbs 5%

Easy Coconut Cookies

Serves: 40

Preparation time: 10 minutes Cooking time: 10 minutes

Ingredients:

- 4 cups unsweetened shredded coconut
- 1/2 cup unsweetened coconut milk
- 1/4 cup erythritol
- 1/4 tsp vanilla

Directions:

1. Add all ingredients to the food processor and process until sticky.
2. Transfer mixture to the large bowl.
3. Make a small ball from mixture and place on a plate.
4. Press each ball lightly into a cookie shape and place in the fridge until firm.
5. Serve and enjoy.

Per Serving: Net Carbs: 0.9g; Calories: 79; Total Fat: 7.1g; Saturated Fat: 6.2g

Protein: 0.9g; Carbs: 2.6g; Fiber: 1.7g; Sugar: 0.9g; Fat 86% / Protein 7% / Carbs 7%

Crunchy Shortbread Cookies

Serves: 6

Preparation time: 10 minutes Cooking time: 10 minutes

Ingredients:

- 1 ¼ cup almond flour
- ½ tsp vanilla
- 3 tbsp butter, softened
- ¼ cup Swerve
- Pinch of salt

Directions:

1. Preheat the oven to 350 F/ 180 C.
2. In a bowl, mix together almond flour, swerve, and salt.
3. Add vanilla and butter and mix until dough is formed.
4. Make cookies from mixture and place on a baking tray.
5. Bake in preheated oven for 10 minutes.
6. Allow to cool completely then serve.

Per Serving: Net Carbs: 2.6g; Calories: 185; Total Fat: 17.4g; Saturated Fat: 4.5g

Protein: 5.1g; Carbs: 5.1g; Fiber: 2.5g; Sugar: 0.9g; Fat 84% / Protein 11% / Carbs 5%

FROZEN DESSERT: BEGINNER

Raspberry Yogurt

Serves: 6

Preparation time: 10 minutes Cooking time: 10 minutes

Ingredients:

- 2 cups plain yogurt
- 5 oz fresh raspberries
- ½ cup erythritol

Directions:

1. Add all ingredients into the blender and blend until smooth.
2. Transfer blended mixture in air-tight container and place in the refrigerator for 40 minutes.
3. Remove yogurt mixture from refrigerator and blend again until smooth.
4. Pour in container and place in the refrigerator for 30 minutes.
5. Serve and enjoy.

Per Serving: Net Carbs: 7g; Calories: 70 Total Fat: 1.9g; Saturated Fat: 0.8g

Protein: 5.1g; Carbs: 8.5g; Fiber: 1.5g; Sugar: 6.8g; Fat 26% / Protein 32% / Carbs 42%

Coconut Butter

Popsicle

Serves: 12

Preparation time: 5 minutes Cooking time: 5 minutes

Ingredients:

- 2 cans unsweetened coconut milk

- 1 tsp liquid stevia

- 1/2 cup peanut butter

Directions:

1. Add all ingredients into the blender and blend until smooth.

2. Pour mixture into the molds and place in the refrigerator for 3 hours or until set.

3. Serve and enjoy.

Per Serving: Net Carbs: 3.1g; Calories: 175 Total Fat: 17.4g; Saturated Fat: 10.7g

Protein: 3.5g; Carbs: 3.7g; Fiber: 0.6g; Sugar: 2.6g; Fat 87% / Protein 7% / Carbs 6%

BREAKFAST RECIPES

Intermediate:

Chicago Italian

Beef Sandwich

All out: 3 hr 40 min

Prep: 20 min

Cook: 3 hr 20 min

Yield: 4 servings

Ingredients

- 4 pounds top round with fat top

- 3 tablespoons Italian flavoring

- 3 tablespoons Worcestershire sauce

- 2 tablespoons salt

- 1 cup garlic, entire cloves

- 2 tablespoons crisp broke dark pepper

- 1 teaspoon cayenne

- 1 tablespoon paprika

- 1 teaspoon red bean stew pieces

- 3 yellow onions, cleaved

- 1/2 cup red wine

- 1 cup hamburger stock

- 2 straight leaves

- 3 tablespoons bacon fat, or canola oil

- 6 sourdough loaf rolls split, toasted

- 1 cup slashed giardiniera vinaigrette vegetables

- 1 cup bumped red sweet peppers

Direction

1. Rub meat with dry fixings, spread and refrigerate for 2 to 3 hours.

2. Preheat broiler to 275 degrees F.

3. Add meat to a simmering skillet with

   bacon fat, include onions and garlic, saute for 15 minutes, deglaze with wine, and include Worcestershire sauce, hamburger stock and straight leaves.

4. Spot simmering skillet in the broiler and cook for 3 hours, revealed, or until a moment read thermometer registers 135 degrees F in focus. Expel, let cool, at that point cut dainty.

5. Cool stock in simmering skillet and evacuate the fat that ascents to the top. Strain.

6. Warm the stock, and include the cut meat. Spot some meat on each toasted move, scoop with some juices and top with giardiniera vegetables and red peppers.

LUNCH RECIPES

Intermediate:

Coconut Bread

Loaves

Nutritional Values:

Calories: 297.5, Total Fat: 14.6 g, Saturated Fat: 2.6 g, Carbs: 25.5 g, Sugars: 0.3 g, Protein:

15.6 g Serves: 4

Ingredients:

- ½ cup Ground Flax Seeds
- ½ tsp Baking Soda
- 1 tsp Baking Powder
- 1 tsp Salt
- 6 Eggs, room temperature
- 1 Tbsp Apple Cider Vinegar
- ½ cup Water
- 1 cup Coconut Flour, sifted

Directions:

1. Ensure that 350F / 175C is the target when preheating your oven. Grease a loaf pan and set aside.

2. Mix together the dry ingredients. Add in the water, eggs, and vinegar and mix well to incorporate.

3. Bake for 40 minutes.

   When baked, leave to cool, slice and enjoy!

SNACKS RECIPES

Rye Crackers

Prep time: 10 minutes Cooking time: 15

minutes

Servings: 10

Nutritional Values:

Calories 80

Total carbs 10.4 g Protein 1.1 g Total

fat 4.3 g

Ingredients:

- 1 cup rye flour
- 2/3 cup bran
- 2 tsp baking powder
- 3 tbsp vegetable oil
- 1 tsp liquid malt extract
- 1 tsp apple vinegar
- 1 cup water
- Salt to taste

Directions:

1. Combine flour with bran, baking powder and salt.
2. Pour in oil, vinegar and malt extract. Mix well.
3. Knead the dough, gradually adding the water.
4. Divide and roll it out with a rolling pin about 0.1 inch thick.
5. Cut out (using a knife or cookie cutter) the crackers of square or rectangle shape.

Bake at 390°F for 12–15 minutes.

THE KETO LUNCH

In this chapter, we'll provide a seven-day menu that you can use for some easy to make but extremely delicious keto lunches.

Monday: Lunch:

Keto Meatballs

Make these ahead of time because these delicious meatballs are freezable. Take a few to work along with some sugar-free marinara sauce and zoodles (zucchini noodles) for a delicious keto lunch.

Variation tip: change the seasonings to make different flavors, like taco or barbecue.

Prep Time: 5 minutes Cook Time: 18 minutes

Servings: 4

What's in it

- Grass-fed ground beef (1 pound)
- Chopped fresh parsley (1.5 t)
- Onion powder (.75 t)
- Garlic powder (.75 t)
- Kosher salt (.75 t)
- Fresh ground black pepper (.5 t)

How it's made

1. Turn oven to 400-degrees F to preheat.
2. Using parchment paper, line a baking sheet.

3. Put beef into a medium-sized glass bowl with other ingredients and mix with hands until just combined. Avoid over-mixing as this will result in tough meatballs.

4. Roll into 8 meatballs and place on the lined baking sheet.

5. Bake for 15-18 minutes until done all the way through.

Net carbs: 3 grams Fat: 17 grams

Protein: 11 grams

Sugars: 2 grams

KETO AT DINNER

Monday: Dinner:

Beef short ribs in

a slow cooker

With a little prep, you will have a hot meal waiting for you at the end of a long day.

Variation tip: serve over diced cauliflower or with celery.

Prep Time: 15 minutes Cook Time: 4 hours

Servings: 4

What's in it

- Boneless short ribs or bone-in (2 pounds)
- Kosher salt (to taste)
- Fresh ground pepper (to taste)
- Extra virgin olive oil (2 T)
- Chopped white onion (1 qty)
- Garlic (3 cloves)
- Bone broth (1 cup)
- Coconut aminos (2 T)
- Tomato paste (2 T)
- Red wine (1.5 cups)

107

How it's made

1. In a large skillet over medium heat, add olive oil. Season meat with salt and pepper. Brown both sides.

2. Add broth and browned ribs to slow cooker

3. Put remaining ingredients into the skillet.

4. Bring to a boil and cook until onions are tender. About 5 minutes.

5. Pour over ribs.

6. Set to 4 to 6 hours on high or 8 to 10 hours on low.

Net carbs: 1 gram

Fat: 63 grams

Protein: 24 grams

Sugars: 1 gram